MICHAEL POLLAN

Food Rules

An Eater's Manual

PENGUIN BOOKS

PENGUIN BOOKS

Published by the Penguin Group
Penguin Books Ltd, 80 Strand, London WC2R 0RL, England
Penguin Group (USA) Inc., 375 Hudson Street, New York, New York 10014, USA
Penguin Group (Canada), 90 Eglinton Avenue East, Suite 700, Toronto, Ontario, Canada M4P 2Y3
(a division of Pearson Penguin Canada Inc.)
Penguin Ireland, 25 St Stephen's Green, Dublin 2, Ireland (a division of Penguin Books Ltd)
Penguin Group (Australia), 250 Camberwell Road, Camberwell, Victoria 3124, Australia
(a division of Pearson Australia Group Pty Ltd)
Penguin Books India Pvt Ltd, 11 Community Centre, Panchsheel Park, New Delhi – 110 017, India
Penguin Group (NZ), 67 Apollo Drive, Rosedale, North Shore 0632, New Zealand
(a division of Pearson New Zealand Ltd)
Penguin Books (South Africa) (Pty) Ltd, 24 Sturdee Avenue,
Rosebank, Johannesburg 2196, South Africa

Penguin Books Ltd, Registered Offices: 80 Strand, London WC2R 0RL, England

www.penguin.com

First published in the United States of America by Penguin Books 2009
First published in Great Britain by Penguin Books 2010

009

978-0-141-04868-0

www.greenpenguin.co.uk

Penguin Books is committed to a sustainable
future for our business, our readers and our planet.
This book is made from Forest Stewardship
Council™ certified paper.

ALWAYS LEARNING   **PEARSON**

PENGUIN BOOKS

FOOD RULES

MICHAEL POLLAN is the author of five previous books, including *In Defence of Food*, a number one *New York Times* bestseller, and *The Omnivore's Dilemma*, which was named one of the ten best books of the year by both the *New York Times* and the *Washington Post*. Both books won the James Beard Award. A long-time contributor to the *New York Times Magazine*, he is also the Knight Professor of Journalism at the University of California at Berkeley.

Contents

For my mother,
who always knew butter was better for you
than margarine

Introduction

Eating in our time has gotten complicated—needlessly so, in my opinion. I will get to the "needlessly" part in a moment, but consider first the complexity that now attends this most basic of creaturely activities. Most of us have come to rely on experts of one kind or another to tell us how to eat—doctors and diet books, media accounts of the latest findings in nutritional science, government advisories and food pyramids, the proliferating health claims on food packages. We may not always heed these experts' advice, but their voices are in our heads every time we order from a menu or wheel down the aisle in the supermarket. Also in our heads today resides an astonishing amount of biochemistry. How odd is it that everybody now has at least a passing acquaintance with words like "antioxidant," "saturated fat," "omega-3 fatty acids," "carbohydrates," "polyphenols," "folic acid," "gluten," and "probiotics"? It's gotten to the point where we don't see *foods* anymore but instead look right through them to the nutrients (good and bad) they contain, and of course to the calories—all these invisible qualities in our food that, properly understood, supposedly hold the secret to eating well.

But for all the scientific and pseudoscientific food baggage we've taken on in recent years, we *still* don't know what we should be eating. Should we worry more about the fats or the carbohydrates? Then what about the "good" fats? Or the "bad" carbohydrates, like high-fructose corn syrup? How much should we be worrying about gluten? What's the deal with artificial sweeteners? Is it really true that this breakfast cereal will improve my son's focus at school or that other cereal will protect me from a heart attack? And when did eating a bowl of breakfast cereal become a therapeutic procedure?

A few years ago, feeling as confused as everyone else, I set out to get to the bottom of a simple question: What should I eat? What do we really know about the links between our diet and our health? I'm not a nutrition expert or a scientist, just a curious journalist hoping to answer a straightforward question for myself and my family.

Most of the time when I embark on such an investigation, it quickly becomes clear that matters are much more complicated and ambiguous—several shades grayer—than I thought going in. Not this time. The deeper I delved into the confused and confusing thicket of nutritional science, sorting through the long-running fats versus carbs wars, the fiber skirmishes and the raging dietary supplement debates, the simpler the picture gradually became. I learned that in fact science knows a lot less about nutrition than you would expect—that in fact nutrition science is, to put it charitably, a very *young* science. It's still trying to figure out exactly what happens in your body when you sip a soda, or what is going on deep in the soul of a carrot to make it so good for you, or why in the world you have so many neurons—brain cells!—in your stomach, of all places. It's a fascinating subject, and someday the field may produce definitive answers to the nutritional questions that concern us, but—as nutritionists themselves will tell you—they're not there yet. Not even close. Nutrition science, which after all only got started less than two hundred years ago, is today approximately where surgery was in the year 1650—very promising, and very interesting to watch, but are you ready to let them operate on you? I think I'll wait awhile.

But if I've learned volumes about all we don't know about nutrition, I've also learned a small number of very important things we *do* know about food and health. This is what I meant when I said the picture got simpler the deeper I went.

There are basically two important things you need to know about the links between diet and health, two facts that are not in dispute. All the contending parties in the nutrition wars agree on them. And, even more important for our purposes, these facts are sturdy enough that we can build a sensible diet upon them. Here they are:

FaCT 1. Populations that eat a so-called Western diet— generally defined as a diet consisting of lots of processed foods and meat, lots of added fat and sugar, lots of refined grains, lots of *every*thing except vegetables, fruits, and whole grains—invariably suffer from high rates of the so-called Western diseases: obesity, type 2 diabetes, cardiovascular disease, and cancer. Virtually all of the obesity and type 2 diabetes, 80 percent of the cardiovascular disease, and more than a third of all cancers can be linked to this diet. Four of the top ten killers in America are chronic diseases linked to this diet. The arguments in nutritional science are not about this well-established link; rather, they are all about identifying the culprit nutrient in the Western diet that might be responsible for chronic diseases. Is it the saturated fat or the refined carbohydrates or the lack of fiber or the transfats or omega-6 fatty acids—or what? The point is that, as eaters (if not as scientists), we know all we need to know to act: This diet, for whatever reason, is the problem.

FaCT 2. Populations eating a remarkably wide range of traditional diets generally don't suffer from these chronic diseases. These diets run the gamut from ones very high in fat (the Inuit in Greenland subsist largely on seal blubber) to ones high in carbohydrate (Central

American Indians subsist largely on maize and beans) to ones very high in protein (Masai tribesmen in Africa subsist chiefly on cattle blood, meat, and milk), to cite three rather extreme examples. But much the same holds true for more mixed traditional diets. What this suggests is that there is no single ideal human diet but that the human omnivore is exquisitely adapted to a wide range of different foods and a variety of different diets. Except, that is, for one: the relatively new (in evolutionary terms) Western diet that most of us now are eating. What an extraordinary achievement for a civilization: to have developed the one diet that reliably makes its people sick! (While it is true that we generally live longer than people used to, or than people in some traditional cultures do, most of our added years owe to gains in infant mortality and child health, not diet.)

There is actually a third, very hopeful fact that flows from these two: People who get off the Western diet see dramatic improvements in their health. We have good research to suggest that the effects of the Western diet can be rolled back, and relatively quickly.* In one analysis, a typical American population that departed even modestly from the Western diet (and lifestyle) could reduce its chances of getting coronary

---

* For a discussion of the research on the Western diet and its alternatives see my previous book, *In Defence of Food* (New York: Penguin Press, 2008). Much of the science behind the rules in this book can be found there.

heart disease by 80 percent, its chances of type 2 diabetes by 90 percent, and its chances of colon cancer by 70 percent.*

Yet, oddly enough, these two (or three) sturdy facts are not the center of our nutritional research or, for that matter, our public health campaigns around diet. Instead, the focus is on identifying *the* evil nutrient in the Western diet so that food manufacturers might tweak their products, thereby leaving the diet undisturbed, or so that pharmaceutical makers might develop and sell us an antidote for it. Why? Well, there's a lot of money in the Western diet. The more you process any food, the more profitable it becomes. The health-care industry makes more money treating chronic diseases (which account for three quarters of the $2 trillion plus we spend each year on health care in this country) than preventing them. So we ignore the elephant in the room and focus instead on good and evil

---

* The diet specified in this analysis is characterized by a low intake of transfats; a high ratio of polyunsaturated fats to saturated fats; a high whole-grain intake; two servings of fish a week; the recommended daily allowance of folic acid; and at least five grams of alcohol a day. The lifestyle changes include not smoking, maintaining a body mass index (BMI) below 25, and thirty minutes a day of exercise. As the author Walter Willett writes, "[T]he potential for disease prevention by modest dietary and lifestyle changes that are readily compatible with life in the 21st century is enormous." "The Pursuit of Optimal Diets: A Progress Report," *Nutritional Genomics: Discovering the Path to Personalized Nutrition*, eds. Jim Kaput and Raymond L. Rodriguez (New York: John Wiley & Sons, 2006).

nutrients, the identities of which seem to change with every new study. But for the Nutritional Industrial Complex this uncertainty is not necessarily a problem, because confusion too is good business: The nutrition experts become indispensable; the food manufacturers can reengineer their products (and health claims) to reflect the latest findings, and those of us in the media who follow these issues have a constant stream of new food and health stories to report. Everyone wins. Except, that is, for us eaters.

As a journalist I fully appreciate the value of widespread public confusion: We're in the explanation business, and if the answers to the questions we explore got too simple, we'd be out of work. Indeed, I had a deeply unsettling moment when, after spending a couple of years researching nutrition for my last book, *In Defense of Food*, I realized that the answer to the supposedly incredibly complicated question of what we should eat wasn't so complicated after all, and in fact could be boiled down to just seven words:

Eat food. Not too much. Mostly plants.

This was the bottom line, and it was satisfying to have found it, a piece of hard ground deep down at the bottom of the swamp of nutrition science: seven words of plain English, no biochemistry degree required. But it was also somewhat alarming, because my publisher was expecting a few thousand more words than that. Fortunately for both of us, I realized that the story of how so simple a question as what to eat had ever gotten so complicated was one worth telling, and that became the focus of that book.

The focus of this book is very different. It is much less about theory, history, and science than it is about our daily lives and practice. In this short, radically pared-down book, I unpack those seven words of advice into a comprehensive set of rules, or personal policies, designed to help you eat real food in moderation and, by doing so, substantially get off the Western diet. The rules are phrased in everyday language; I deliberately avoid the vocabulary of nutrition or biochemistry, though in most cases there is scientific research to back them up.

This book is not antiscience. To the contrary, in researching it and vetting these rules I have made good use of science and scientists. But I am skeptical of a lot of what passes for nutritional science, and I believe that there are other sources of wisdom in the world and other vocabularies in which to talk intelligently about food. Human beings ate well and kept themselves healthy for millennia before nutritional science came along to tell us how to do it; it is entirely possible to eat healthily without knowing what an antioxidant is.

So whom did we rely on before the scientists (and, in turn, governments, public health organizations, and food marketers) began telling us how to eat? We relied of course on our mothers and grandmothers and more distant ancestors, which is another way of saying, on tradition and culture. We know there is a deep reservoir of food wisdom out there, or else humans would not have survived and prospered to the extent we have. This dietary wisdom is the distillation of an evolutionary process involving many people in many places figuring out what keeps people healthy (and what doesn't), and passing that knowledge down in the form of food habits and combinations, manners and rules and taboos, and everyday and seasonal practices, as well as memorable sayings and adages. Are these traditions infallible? No. There are plenty of old wives' tales about food that on inspection turn out to be little more than superstitions. But much of this food wisdom is worth preserving and reviving and heeding. That is exactly what this book aims to do.

Food Rules distills this body of wisdom into sixty-four simple rules for eating healthily and happily. The rules are framed in terms of culture rather than science, though in many cases science has confirmed what culture has long known; not surprisingly, these two different vocabularies, or ways of knowing, often come to the same conclusion (as when scientists recently confirmed that the traditional practice of eating tomatoes with olive oil is good for you, because the lycopene in the tomatoes is soluble in oil, making it easier for your body to absorb). I have also avoided talking much about nutrients, not because they aren't important, but because focusing relentlessly on nutrients obscures other, more important truths about food.

Foods are more than the sum of their nutrient parts, and those nutrients work together in ways that are still only dimly understood. It may be that the degree to which a food is processed gives us a more important key to its healthfulness: Not only can processing remove nutrients and add toxic chemicals, but it makes food more readily absorbable, which can be a problem for our insulin and fat metabolism. Also, the plastics in which processed foods are typically packaged can present a further risk to our health. This is why many of the rules in this book are designed to help you avoid heavily processed foods—which I prefer to call "edible foodlike substances."

Most of these rules I wrote, but many of them have no single author. They are pieces of food culture, sometimes ancient, that deserve our attention, because they can help us. I've collected these adages about eating from a wide variety of sources. (The older sayings appear in quotes.) I consulted folklorists and anthropologists, doctors, nurses, nutritionists, and dietitians, as well as a large number of mothers, grandmothers, and great-grandmothers. I solicited food rules from my readers and from audiences at conferences and speeches on three continents; I publicized a Web address where people could e-mail rules they had heard from their parents or others and had found personally helpful. A single request for rules that I posted on the *New York Times*'s "Well" blog resulted in twenty-five hundred suggestions. Not all of them made a whole lot of sense ("One meat per pizza" is probably not a surefire prescription for good health), but many of them did, and several are included here. Thank you to all who contributed to the project. Taken together, these rules comprise a kind of choral voice of popular food wisdom. My job has been not to create that wisdom so much as to curate it and vet it. My wager is that that voice has as much or more to teach us, and to help us right our relationship to food, than the voices of science and industry and government.

The sixty-four rules here are each accompanied by a paragraph or two of explanation, except for a few that are self-explanatory. There is no need to learn or memorize them all, because many will take you to the same place. For example, rule number 11 ("Avoid foods you see advertised on television") and rule number 7 ("Avoid food products containing ingredients that a third-grader cannot pronounce") are both designed to keep more or less the same highly processed foodlike products out of your cart. My hope is that a handful of these rules will prove sufficiently sticky, or memorable, that they will become second nature to you—something you do, or don't do, without giving it a thought.

While I call them rules, I think of them less as hard-and-fast laws than as personal policies. Policies are useful tools. Instead of prescribing highly specific behaviors, they supply us with broad guidelines that should make everyday decision making easier and swifter. Armed with a general policy, like rule number

36 ("Don't eat breakfast cereals that change the color of the milk"), you'll find you won't have to waste as much time reading ingredients labels and making decisions standing in the cereal aisle. Think of these food policies as little algorithms designed to simplify your eating life. Adopt whichever ones stick and work best for you.

But do be sure to adopt at least one from each of the three sections, because each section deals with a different dimension of your eating life. The first section is designed to help you "eat food," which in the modern supermarket turns out to be a lot more difficult than you would think. These rules offer screens or filters to help you tell the real food from the edible foodlike substances you want to avoid. The second section, subtitled "Mostly plants," offers rules to help you choose among real foods. And the third, subtitled "Not too much," deals with *how* rather than *what* to eat and offers a series of policies designed to foster some simple everyday habits that will help you moderate your eating *and* enjoy it more. If those two goals sound contradictory, well, you haven't dipped into this book yet.

PART I

What should I eat?

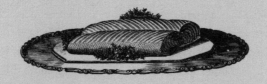

(Eat food.)

The rules in this section will help you to distinguish real foods—the plants, animals, and fungi people have been eating for generations—from the highly processed products of modern food science that, increasingly, have come to dominate the American food marketplace and diet. Each rule proposes a different filter for separating the one from the other, but they all share a common aim, which is to help you keep the unhealthy stuff out of your shopping cart.

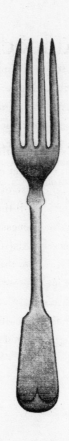

Eat food.

These days this is easier said than done, especially when seventeen thousand new products show up in the supermarket each year, all vying for your food dollar. But most of these items don't deserve to be called food—I call them edible foodlike substances. They're highly processed concoctions designed by food scientists, consisting mostly of ingredients derived from corn and soy that no normal person keeps in the pantry, and they contain chemical additives with which the human body has not been long acquainted. Today much of the challenge of eating well comes down to choosing real food and avoiding these industrial novelties.

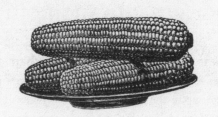

2

Don't eat anything your great-grandmother wouldn't recognize as food.

Imagine your great-grandmother (or grandmother, depending on your age) at your side as you roll down the aisles of the supermarket. You're standing together in front of the dairy case. She picks up a package of Go-GURT Portable Yogurt tubes—and hasn't a clue what this plastic cylinder of colored and flavored gel could possibly be. Is it a food or is it toothpaste? There are now thousands of foodish products in the supermarket that our ancestors simply wouldn't recognize as food. The reasons to avoid eating such complicated food products are many, and go beyond the various chemical additives and corn and soy derivatives they contain, or the plastics in which they are typically packaged, some of which are probably toxic. Today foods are processed in ways specifically designed to get us to buy and eat more by pushing our evolutionary buttons—our inborn preferences for sweetness and fat and salt. These tastes are difficult to find in nature but cheap and easy for the food scientist to deploy, with the result that food processing induces us to consume much more of these rarities than is good for us. The great-grandma rule will help keep most of these items out of your cart.

Note: If your great-grandmother was a terrible cook or eater, you can substitute someone else's grandmother—a Sicilian or French one works particularly well.

The next several rules refine this strategy by helping you navigate the treacherous landscape of the ingredients label.

3

Avoid food products containing ingredients that no ordinary human would keep in the pantry.

Ethoxylated diglycerides? Cellulose? Xanthan gum? Calcium propionate? Ammonium sulfate? If you wouldn't cook with them yourself, why let others use these ingredients to cook for you? The food scientists' chemistry set is designed to extend shelf life, make old food look fresher and more appetizing than it really is, and get you to eat more. Whether or not any of these additives pose a proven hazard to your health, many of them haven't been eaten by humans for very long, so they are best avoided.

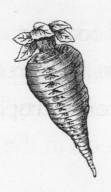

Avoid food products that contain high-fructose corn syrup.

Not because high-fructose corn syrup (HFCS) is any worse for you than sugar, but because it is, like many of the other unfamiliar ingredients in packaged foods, a reliable marker for a food product that has been highly processed. Also, high-fructose corn syrup is being added to hundreds of foods that have not traditionally been sweetened—breads, condiments, and many snack foods—so if you avoid products that contain it, you will cut down on your sugar intake. But don't fall for the food industry's latest scam: products reformulated to contain "no HFCS" or "real cane sugar." These claims imply these foods are somehow healthier, but they're not. Sugar is sugar.

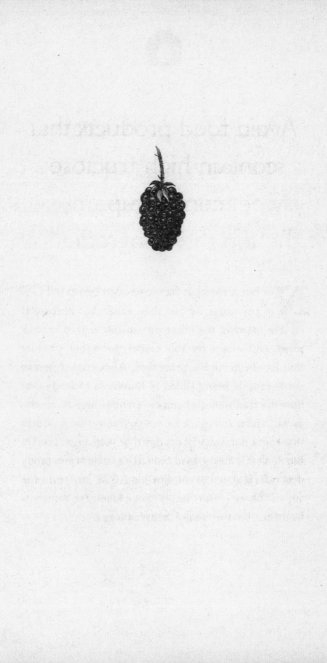

5

Avoid foods that have some form of sugar (or sweetener) listed among the top three ingredients.

Labels list ingredients by weight, and any product that has more sugar than other ingredients has too much sugar. (For an exception to this rule, see rule 60, regarding special occasion foods.) Complicating matters is the fact that, thanks to food science, there are now some forty types of sugar used in processed food, including barley malt, beet sugar, brown rice syrup, cane juice, corn sweetener, dextrin, dextrose, fructo-oligosaccharides, fruit juice concentrate, glucose, sucrose, invert sugar, polydextrose, sucrose, turbinado sugar, and so on. To repeat: Sugar is sugar. And organic sugar is sugar too. As for noncaloric sweeteners such as aspartame or Splenda, research (in both humans and animals) suggests that switching to artificial sweeteners does not lead to weight loss, for reasons not yet well understood. But it may be that deceiving the brain with the reward of sweetness stimulates a craving for even more sweetness.

6

Avoid food products that contain more than five ingredients.

The specific number you adopt is arbitrary, but the more ingredients in a packaged food, the more highly processed it probably is. Note 1: A long list of ingredients in a recipe is not the same thing; that's fine. Note 2: Some products now boast, somewhat deceptively, about their short ingredient lists. Häagen-Dazs has a new line of ice cream called "five." Great—but it's still ice cream. Same goes for the three-ingredient Tostitos corn chips advertised by Frito-Lay—okay, but they're still corn chips. In such cases, apply rule 60 for dealing with treats and special occasion foods.

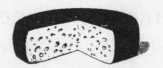

Avoid food products containing ingredients that a third-grader cannot pronounce.

Basically the same idea, different mnemonic. Keep it simple!

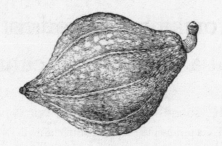

Avoid food products that make health claims.

This sounds counterintuitive, but consider: For a product to carry a health claim on its package, it must first have a package, so right off the bat it's more likely to be a processed rather than a whole food. Then, only the big food manufacturers have the wherewithal to secure FDA-approved health claims for their products and then trumpet them to the world. Generally, it is the products of modern food science that make the boldest health claims, and these are often founded on incomplete and often bad science. Don't forget that margarine, one of the first industrial foods to claim it was more healthful than the traditional food it replaced, turned out to contain transfats that give people heart attacks. The healthiest food in the supermarket—the fresh produce—doesn't boast about its healthfulness, because the growers don't have the budget or the packaging. Don't take the silence of the yams as a sign they have nothing valuable to say about your health.

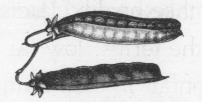

Avoid food products with the wordoid "lite" or the terms "low-fat" or "nonfat" in their names.

The forty-year-old campaign to create low- and nonfat versions of traditional foods has been a failure: We've gotten fat on low-fat products. Why? Because removing the fat from foods doesn't necessarily make them nonfattening. Carbohydrates can also make you fat, and many low- and nonfat foods boost the sugars to make up for the loss of flavor. Also, by demonizing one nutrient—fat—we inevitably give a free pass to another, supposedly "good," nutrient—carbohydrates in this case—and then proceed to eat too much of that instead. Since the low-fat campaign began in the late 1970s, Americans actually have been eating more than 500 additional calories per day, most of them in the form of refined carbohydrates like sugar.

The result: The average male is seventeen pounds heavier and the average female nineteen pounds heavier than in the late 1970s. You're better off eating the real thing in moderation than bingeing on "lite" food products packed with sugars and salt.

Avoid foods that
are pretending to be
something they are not.

Imitation butter—aka margarine—is the classic example. To make something like nonfat cream cheese that contains neither cream nor cheese requires an extreme degree of processing; such products should be labeled as imitations and avoided. The same rule applies to soy-based mock meats, artificial sweeteners, and fake fats and starches.

Avoid foods you see advertised on television.

Food marketers are ingenious at turning criticisms of their products—and rules like these—into new ways to sell slightly different versions of the same processed foods: They simply reformulate (to be low-fat, have no HFCS or transfats, or to contain fewer ingredients) and then boast about their implied healthfulness, whether the boast is meaningful or not. The best way to escape these marketing ploys is to tune out the marketing itself, by refusing to buy heavily promoted foods. Only the biggest food manufacturers can afford to advertise their products on television: More than two thirds of food advertising is spent promoting processed foods (and alcohol), so if you avoid products with big ad budgets, you'll automatically be avoiding edible foodlike substances. As for the 5 percent of food ads that promote whole foods (the prune or walnut growers or the beef ranchers), common sense will, one hopes, keep you from tarring them with the same brush—these are the exceptions that prove the rule.

Bogus health claims and faulty food science have made supermarkets particularly treacherous places to shop for real food, which suggests the next two rules.

14

Eat foods made from ingredients that you can picture in their raw state or growing in nature.

Read the ingredients on a package of Twinkies or Pringles and imagine what those ingredients actually look like raw or in the places where they grow: You can't do it. This rule will keep all sorts of chemicals and foodlike substances out of your diet.

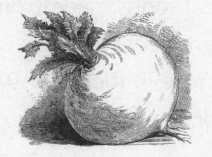

Get out of the supermarket whenever you can.

You won't find any high-fructose corn syrup at the farmers' market. You also won't find any elaborately processed food products, any packages with long lists of unpronounceable ingredients or dubious health claims, anything microwaveable, or, perhaps best of all, any old food from far away. What you will find are fresh, whole foods harvested at the peak of their taste and nutritional quality—precisely the kind your great-grandmother, or even your Neolithic ancestors, would easily recognize as food. The kind that is alive and eventually will rot.

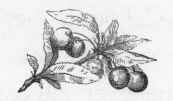

Shop the peripheries of the supermarket and stay out of the middle.

Most supermarkets are laid out the same way: Processed food products dominate the center aisles of the store, while the cases of mostly fresh food—produce, meat and fish, dairy—line the walls. If you keep to the edges of the store you'll be much more likely to wind up with real food in your shopping cart. This strategy is not foolproof, however, since things like high-fructose corn syrup have crept into the dairy case under the cover of flavored yogurts and the like.

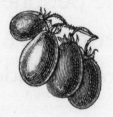

Eat only foods that will eventually rot.

What does it mean for food to "go bad"? It usually means that the fungi and bacteria and insects and rodents with whom we compete for nutrients and calories have gotten to it before we did. Food processing began as a way to extend the shelf life of food by protecting it from these competitors. This is often accomplished by making the food less appealing to them, by removing nutrients from it that attract competitors, or by removing other nutrients likely to turn rancid, like omega-3 fatty acids. The more processed a food is, the longer the shelf life, and the less nutritious it typically is. Real food is alive—and therefore it should eventually die. (There are a few exceptions to this rule: For example, honey has a shelf life measured in centuries.) Note: Most of the immortal foodlike substances in the supermarket are found in the middle aisles.

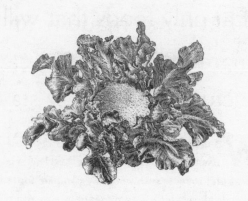

Eat only foods that have been cooked by humans.

If you're going to let others cook for you, you're much better off if they are other humans, rather than corporations. In general, corporations cook with too much salt, fat, and sugar, as well as with preservatives, colorings, and other biological novelties. They also aim for immortality in their food products. Note: While it is true that professional chefs are generally humans, they often cook with large amounts of salt, fat, and sugar too, so treat restaurant meals as special occasions.

Following are a few useful variants on the human-cooked-food rule.

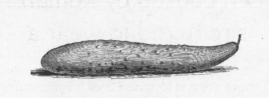

18

Don't ingest foods made
in places where everyone
is required to wear a
surgical cap.

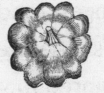

If it came from a plant,
eat it; if it was made in
a plant, don't.

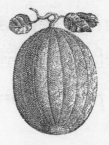

20

It's not food if it arrived
through the window
of your car.

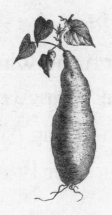

21

It's not food if it's called
by the same name in
every language.
(Think Big Mac,
Cheetos, or Pringles.)

PART II

What kind of food should I eat?

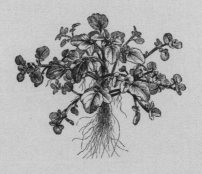

(Mostly plants.)

If you follow the rules offered thus far you will be eating real, whole food most of the time—the simple key to a healthy diet. Beyond that, you have a great many options. One lesson that can be drawn from the striking diversity of traditional diets people have lived on around the world is that it is possible to nourish ourselves from an astonishing range of foods—so long as they really are foods. There have been, and can be, healthy high-fat and healthy low-fat diets, but they have always been diets built around whole foods. Yet there are some whole foods that are better for us than others, and some ways of producing them and then combining them in meals that can make a difference. So the rules in this section propose a handful of personal policies regarding what to eat, above and beyond "food."

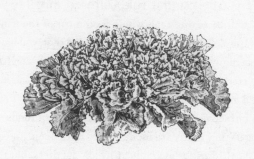

Eat mostly plants, especially leaves.

Scientists may disagree on what's so good about plants—the antioxidants? the fiber? the omega-3 fatty acids?—but they do agree that they're probably really good for you and certainly can't hurt. There are scores of studies demonstrating that a diet rich in vegetables and fruits reduces the risk of dying from all the Western diseases; in countries where people eat a pound or more of vegetables and fruits a day, the rate of cancer is half what it is in the United States. Also, by eating a diet that is primarily plant based, you'll be consuming far fewer calories, since plant foods—with the exception of seeds, including grains and nuts—are typically less "energy dense" than the other things you eat. (And consuming fewer calories protects against many chronic diseases.) Vegetarians are notably healthier than carnivores, and they live longer.

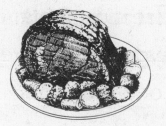

Treat meat as a flavoring or special occasion food.

While it's true that vegetarians are generally healthier than carnivores, that doesn't mean you need to eliminate meat from your diet if you like it. Meat, which humans have been eating and relishing for a very long time, is nourishing food, which is why I suggest "mostly" plants, not "only." It turns out that near vegetarians, or "flexitarians"—people who eat meat a couple of times a week—are just as healthy as vegetarians. But the average American eats meat as part of two or even three meals a day—more than half a pound per person per day—and there is evidence that the more meat there is in your diet—red meat in particular—the greater your risk of heart disease and cancer. Why? It could be its saturated fat, or its specific type of protein, or the simple fact that all that meat is pushing plants off the plate. Consider swapping the traditional portion sizes: Instead of an eight-ounce steak and a four-ounce portion of vegetables, serve four ounces of beef and eight ounces of veggies. Thomas Jefferson was probably onto something when he recommended a mostly plant-based diet that uses meat chiefly as a "flavor principle."

"Eating what stands on one leg [mushrooms and plant foods] is better than eating what stands on two legs [fowl], which is better than eating what stands on four legs [cows, pigs, and other mammals]."

This Chinese proverb offers a good summary of traditional wisdom regarding the relative healthfulness of different kinds of food, though it inexplicably leaves out the very healthful and entirely legless fish.

Eat your colors.

The idea that a healthy plate of food will feature several different colors is a good example of an old wives' tale about food that turns out to be good science too. The colors of many vegetables reflect the different antioxidant phytochemicals they contain— anthocyanins, polyphenols, flavonoids, carotenoids. Many of these chemicals help protect against chronic diseases, but each in a slightly different way, so the best protection comes from a diet containing as many different phytochemicals as possible.

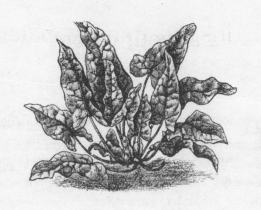

Drink the spinach water.

Another bit of traditional wisdom with good science behind it: The water in which vegetables are cooked is rich in vitamins and other healthful plant chemicals. Save it for soup or add it to sauces.

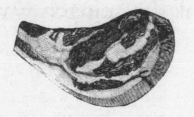

Eat animals that have themselves eaten well.

The diet of the animals we eat strongly influences the nutritional quality, and healthfulness, of the food we get from them, whether it is meat or milk or eggs. This should be self-evident, yet it is a truth routinely overlooked by the industrial food chain in its quest to produce vast quantities of cheap animal protein. That quest has changed the diet of most of our food animals in ways that have often damaged their health and healthfulness. We feed animals a high-energy diet of grain to make them grow quickly, even in the case of ruminants that have evolved to eat grass. But even food animals that can tolerate grain are much healthier when they have access to green plants—and so, it turns out, are their meat and eggs. The food from these animals will contain much healthier types of fat (more omega-3s, less omega-6s) as well as appreciably higher levels of vitamins and antioxidants. (For the same reason, meat from wild animals is particularly nutritious; see rule 31.) It's worth looking for pastured animal foods in the market—and paying the premium prices they typically command if you can.

If you have the space, buy a freezer.

When you find a good source of pastured meat, you'll want to buy it in quantity. Buying meat in bulk—a quarter of a steer, say, or a whole hog—is one way to eat well on a budget. Dedicated freezers are surprisingly inexpensive to buy and to operate, because they aren't opened nearly as often as the one in your refrigerator. A freezer will also enable you to put up food from the farmers' market, and encourage you to buy produce in bulk at the height of its season, when it will be most abundant—and therefore cheapest. And freezing does not significantly diminish the nutritional value of produce.

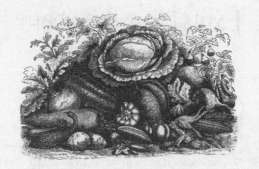

Eat like an omnivore.

Whether or not you eat any animal foods, it's a good idea to try to add some new species, and not just new foods, to your diet—that is, new kinds of plants, animals, and fungi. The dazzling diversity of food products on offer in the supermarket is deceptive, because so many of them are made from the same small handful of plant species, and most of those—the corn and soy and wheat—are seeds rather than leaves. The greater the diversity of species you eat, the more likely you are to cover all your nutritional bases.

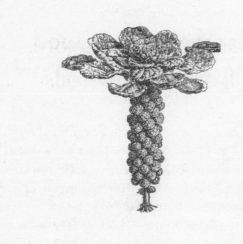

Eat well-grown food
from healthy soil.

It would have been easier to say "eat organic," and it is true that food certified organic is usually well grown in relatively healthy soil—soil nourished by organic matter rather than chemical fertilizers. (It also will contain little or no residue from synthetic pesticides or pharmaceuticals.) Yet there are exceptional farmers and ranchers in America who for one reason or another are not certified organic, and the excellent food they grow should not be overlooked. (And just because a food is labeled organic does not mean it's good for you: Organic soda is still soda—a large quantity of utterly empty calories.)

We now have a body of research supporting the hypothesis, first advanced by organic pioneers Sir Albert Howard and J. I. Rodale, that soils rich in organic matter produce more nutritious food: that is, food with higher levels of antioxidants, flavonoids, vitamins, and minerals. Of course, after a few days riding cross-country in a truck, the nutritional quality of any kind of produce will deteriorate, so ideally you want to eat food that is both organic *and* local.

Eat wild foods
when you can.

Two of the most nutritious plants in the world —lamb's quarters and purslane—are weeds, and some of the healthiest traditional diets, like the Mediterranean, make frequent use of wild greens. The fields and forests are crowded with plants containing higher levels of various phytochemicals than their domesticated cousins. Why? Because these plants have to defend themselves against pests and diseases without any help from us, and because historically we've tended to select and breed crop plants for sweetness; many of the defensive compounds plants produce are bitter. We also breed for shelf life, and so have unwittingly selected for plants with low levels of omega-3 fatty acids, since these fats quickly oxidize—turn rancid. Wild animals and fish too are worth adding to your diet when you have the opportunity. Wild game generally has less saturated and more healthy fats than domesticated animals, because most of these wild animals themselves eat a diverse diet of plants rather than grain (see rule 27).

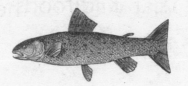

Don't overlook the oily little fishes.

Wild fish are among the healthiest things you can eat, yet many wild fish stocks are on the verge of collapse because of overfishing. Avoid big fish at the top of the marine food chain—tuna, swordfish, shark—because they're endangered, and because they often contain high levels of mercury. Fortunately, a few of the most nutritious wild fish species, including mackerel, sardines, and anchovies, are well managed, and in some cases are even abundant. Those oily little fish are particularly good choices. According to a Dutch proverb, "A land with lots of herring can get along with few doctors."

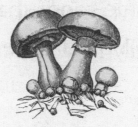

Eat some foods that have been predigested by bacteria or fungi.

Many traditional cultures swear by the health benefits of fermented foods—foods that have been transformed by live microorganisms, such as yogurt, sauerkraut, soy sauce, kimchi, and sourdough bread. These foods can be a good source of vitamin B_{12}, an essential nutrient you can't get from plants. (B_{12} is produced by animals and bacteria.) Many fermented foods also contain probiotics—beneficial bacteria that research suggests improve the function of the digestive and immune systems and, according to some studies, help reduce allergic reactions and inflammation.

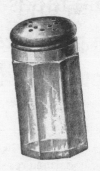

Sweeten and salt your food yourself.

Whether soups or cereals or soft drinks, foods and beverages that have been prepared by corporations contain far higher levels of salt and sugar than any ordinary human would ever add—even a child. By sweetening and salting these foods yourself, you'll make them to your taste, and you will find you're consuming a fraction as much sugar and salt as you otherwise would.

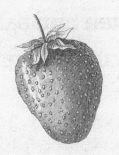

Eat sweet foods as you find them in nature.

In nature, sugars almost always come packaged with fiber, which slows their absorption and gives you a sense of satiety before you've ingested too many calories. That's why you're always better off eating the fruit rather than drinking its juice. (In general, calories taken in liquid form are more fattening because they don't make us feel full. Humans are one of the very few mammals that obtain calories from liquids after weaning.) So don't drink your sweets, and remember: There is no such thing as a healthy soda.

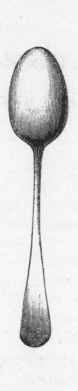

Don't eat breakfast cereals that change the color of the milk.

This should go without saying. Such cereals are highly processed and full of refined carbohydrates as well as chemical additives.

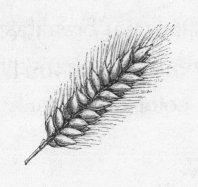

"The whiter the bread, the sooner you'll be dead."

This rather blunt bit of cross-cultural grand-motherly advice (passed down from both Jewish and Italian grandmothers) suggests that the health risks of white flour have been popularly recognized for many years. As far as the body is concerned, white flour is not much different from sugar. Unless supple-mented, it offers none of the good things (fiber, B vita-mins, healthy fats) in whole grains—it's little more than a shot of glucose. Large spikes of glucose are inflammatory and wreak havoc on our insulin metab-olism. Eat whole grains and minimize your consump-tion of white flour. Recent research indicates that the grandmothers who lived by this rule were right: People who eat lots of whole grains tend to be healthier and to live longer.

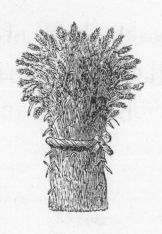

Favor the kinds of oils and grains that have traditionally been stone-ground.

When grindstones were the only way to refine flour and oil, flour and oil were generally more nutritious. In the case of grain, more of the germ and fiber remains when it is ground on a stone; you can't get white flour from a stone. The nutritional benefits of whole grains are impressive: fiber; the full range of B vitamins; and healthy oils, all of which are sacrificed when the grain is refined on modern roller mills (as mentioned, highly refined flours are little different from sugar). And the newer oils that are extracted by modern chemical means tend to have less favorable fatty acid profiles and more additives than olive, sesame, palm fruit, and peanut oils that have been obtained the old-fashioned way.

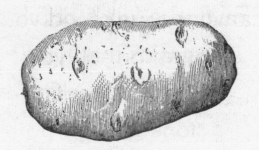

Eat all the junk food you want as long as you cook it yourself.

There is nothing wrong with eating sweets, fried foods, pastries, even drinking a soda every now and then, but food manufacturers have made eating these formerly expensive and hard-to-make treats so cheap and easy that we're eating them every day. The french fry did not become America's most popular vegetable until industry took over the jobs of washing, peeling, cutting, and frying the potatoes— and cleaning up the mess. If you made all the french fries you ate, you would eat them much less often, if only because they're so much work. The same holds true for fried chicken, chips, cakes, pies, and ice cream. Enjoy these treats as often as you're willing to prepare them—chances are good it won't be every day.

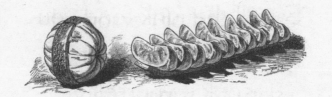

Be the kind of person who takes supplements—then skip the supplements.

We know that people who take supplements are generally healthier than the rest of us, and we also know that in controlled studies most of the supplements they take don't appear to be effective. How can this be? Supplement takers are healthy for reasons that have nothing to do with the pills. They're typically more health conscious, better educated, and more affluent. They're also more likely to exercise and eat whole grains. So to the extent you can, be the *kind* of person who would take supplements, and then save your money. (There are exceptions to this rule, for people who have a specific nutrient deficiency or are older than fifty. As we age, our need for antioxidants increases while our body's ability to absorb them from the diet declines. And if you don't eat much fish, it couldn't hurt to take a fish oil supplement too.)

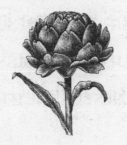

41

Eat more like the French. Or the Japanese. Or the Italians. Or the Greeks.

People who eat according to the rules of a traditional food culture are generally healthier than those of us eating a modern Western diet of processed foods. Any traditional diet will do: If it were not a healthy diet, the people who follow it wouldn't still be around. True, food cultures are embedded in societies and economies and ecologies, and some of them travel better than others, Inuit not so well as Italian. In borrowing from a food culture, pay attention to *how* a culture eats as well as to what it eats. In the case of the French paradox, for example, it may not be the dietary nutrients that keep the French healthy (lots of saturated fat and white flour?!) as much as their food habits: small portions eaten at leisurely communal meals; no second helpings or snacking. Pay attention, too, to the combinations of foods in traditional cultures: In Latin

America, corn is traditionally cooked with lime and eaten with beans; what would otherwise be a nutritionally deficient staple becomes the basis of a healthy, balanced diet. (The beans supply amino acids lacking in corn, and the lime makes niacin available.) Cultures that took corn from Latin America without the beans or the lime wound up with serious nutritional deficiencies such as pellagra. Traditional diets are more than the sum of their food parts.

42

Regard
nontraditional foods
with skepticism.

I nnovation is always interesting, but when it comes to food, it pays to approach new creations with caution. If diets are the products of an evolutionary process in which groups of people adapt to the plants, animals, and fungi a particular place has to offer, then a novel food or culinary innovation resembles a mutation: It *might* represent an evolutionary improvement, but chances are it doesn't. Soy products offer a good case in point. People have been eating soy in the form of tofu, soy sauce, and tempeh for many generations, but today we're eating novelties like "soy protein isolate," "soy isoflavones," and "textured vegetable protein" from soy and partially hydrogenated soy oils, and there are questions about the healthfulness of these new food products. As a senior FDA scientist has written, "Confidence that soy products are safe is clearly based more on belief than hard data."* Until we have that data, you're probably better off eating soy prepared in the traditional Asian manner than according to the novel recipes dreamed up by food scientists.

* D. M. Sheehan, "Herbal Medicines, Phytoestrogens, and Toxicity: Risk: Benefit Considerations," *Proceedings of the Society for Experimental Biology and Medicine* 217 (1998): 379–85.

Have a glass of wine with dinner.

Wine may not be the magic bullet in the French or Mediterranean diet, but it does seem to be an integral part of these dietary patterns. There is now considerable scientific evidence for the health benefits of alcohol to go with a few centuries of traditional belief and anecdotal evidence. Mindful of the social and health effects of alcoholism, public health authorities are loath to recommend drinking, but the fact is that people who drink moderately and regularly live longer and suffer considerably less heart disease than teetotalers. Alcohol of any kind appears to reduce the risk of heart disease, but the polyphenols in red wine (resveratrol in particular) may have unique protective qualities. Most experts recommend no more than two drinks a day for men, one for women. Also, the health benefits of alcohol may depend as much on the pattern of drinking as on the amount: Drinking a little every day is better than drinking a lot on the weekends, and drinking with food is better than drinking without it. Someday science may figure out the complex synergies at work in a traditional diet that includes wine, but until then we can marvel at its accumulated wisdom—and raise a glass to paradox.

PART III

How should I eat?

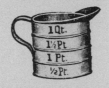

(Not too much.)

The rules in the previous two sections deal primarily with questions about what to eat; the ones in this section deal with something a bit more elusive but no less important: the set of manners, eating habits, taboos, and unspoken guidelines that together govern a person's (and a culture's) relationship to food and eating. *How* you eat may have as much bearing on your health (and your weight) as *what* you eat.

This may well be the deeper lesson of the so-called French paradox: the mystery (at least to nutritionists) of a population that eats all sorts of supposedly lethal fatty foods, and washes them down with red wine, but which is nevertheless healthier, slimmer, and slightly longer lived than we are. What nutritionists fail to see in the French is a people with a completely different relationship to food than we have. They seldom snack, eat small portions from small plates, don't go back for second helpings, and eat most of their food at long, leisurely meals shared with other people. The rules governing these behaviors may matter more than any magic nutrient in their diet.

The rules in this section are designed to foster a healthier relationship to food, whatever it is you're eating.

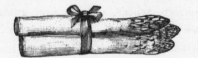

Pay more,
eat less.

With food, as with so many things, you get what you pay for. There is also a trade-off between quality and quantity, and a person's "food experience"—a meal's duration or quotient of pleasure—does not necessarily correlate with the number of calories consumed. The American food system has for many years devoted its energies to increasing quantity and reducing price rather than to improving quality. There's no escaping the fact that better food—measured by taste or nutritional quality (which often correspond)—costs more, because it has been grown or raised less intensively and with more care. Not everyone can afford to eat well in America, which is a literal shame, but most of us can: Americans spend less than 10 percent of their income on food, less than the citizens of any other nation. As the cost of food in America has declined, in terms of both price and the effort required to put it on the table, we have been eating much more (and spending more on health care). If you spend more for better food, you'll probably eat less of it, and treat it with more care. And if that higher-quality food tastes better, you will need less of it to feel satisfied. Choose quality over quantity, food experience over mere calories. Or as grandmothers used to say, "Better to pay the grocer than the doctor."

... Eat less.

This is probably the most unwelcome advice of all, but in fact the scientific case for eating a lot less than we currently do—regardless of whether you are overweight—is compelling. "Calorie restriction" has repeatedly been shown to slow aging in animals, and many researchers believe it offers the single strongest link between diet and cancer prevention. We eat much more than our bodies need to be healthy, and the excess wreaks havoc—and not just on our weight. But we are not the first people in history to grapple with the special challenges posed by food abundance, and previous cultures have devised various ways to promote the idea of moderation. The rules that follow offer a few proven strategies.

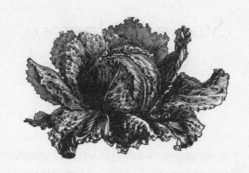

Stop eating before you're full.

Nowadays we think it is normal and right to eat until you are full, but many cultures specifically advise stopping well before that point is reached. The Japanese have a saying—*hara hachi bu*—counseling people to stop eating when they are 80 percent full. The Ayurvedic tradition in India advises eating until you are 75 percent full; the Chinese specify 70 percent, and the prophet Muhammad described a full belly as one that contained ⅓ food and ⅓ liquid—and ⅓ air, i.e., nothing. (Note the relatively narrow range specified in all this advice: somewhere between 67 and 80 percent of capacity. Take your pick.) There's also a German expression that says: "You need to tie off the sack before it gets completely full." And how many of us have grandparents who talk of "leaving the table a little bit hungry"? Here again the French may have something to teach us. To say "I'm hungry" in French you say "J'ai faim"—"I have hunger"—and when you are finished,

you do not say that you are full, but "Je n'ai plus faim"—
"I have no more hunger." That is a completely different
way of thinking about satiety. So: Ask yourself not, Am
I full? but, Is my hunger gone? That moment will arrive
several bites sooner.

Eat when you are hungry, not when you are bored.

For many of us, eating has surprisingly little to do with hunger. We eat out of boredom, for entertainment, to comfort or reward ourselves. Try to be aware of *why* you're eating, and ask yourself if you're really hungry—before you eat and then again along the way. (One old wives' test: If you're not hungry enough to eat an apple, then you're not hungry.) Food is a costly antidepressant.

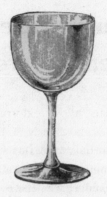

Consult your gut.

Most of us allow external, and usually visual, cues to determine how much we eat. The larger the portion, for example, the more we eat; the bigger the container, the more we pour. As in so many areas of modern life, the culture of food has become a culture of the eye. But when it comes to food, it pays to cultivate the other senses, which often provide more useful and accurate information. It can take twenty minutes before your brain gets the word that your belly is full; that means that if you take less than twenty minutes to finish a meal, the sensation of satiety will arrive too late to be of any use. So slow down and pay attention to what your body—and not just your sense of sight—is telling you. This is what your grandparents were getting at with the adage "Your eyes are bigger than your stomach."

Cauliflower

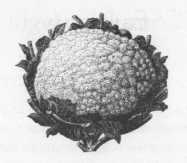

Eat slowly.

Not just so you'll be more likely to know when to stop. Eat slowly enough to savor your food; you'll need less of it to feel satisfied. If it is a food experience rather than mere calories you're after, the slower you eat, the more of an experience you will have. There is an Indian proverb that gets at this idea: "Drink your food, chew your drink." In other words, eat slowly enough, and chew thoroughly enough, to liquefy your food, and move your drink around in your mouth to thoroughly taste it before swallowing. The recommendation sounds a bit clinical perhaps, but try following it at least to the point of fully appreciating what's in your mouth. Another strategy, encoded in a table manner that's been all but forgotten: "Put down your fork between bites."

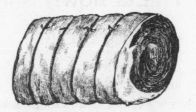

"The banquet is in
the first bite."

Taking this adage to heart will help you enjoy your food and eat more slowly. No other bite will taste as good as the first, and every subsequent bite will progressively diminish in satisfaction. Economists call this the law of diminishing marginal utility, and it argues for savoring the first few bites and stopping sooner than you otherwise might. For as you go on, you'll be getting more calories, but not necessarily more pleasure.

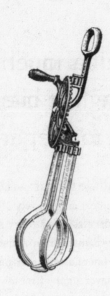

Spend as much time enjoying the meal as it took to prepare it.

This is a pretty good metric that honors the cook for the care you or he or she has put into the meal at the same time that it helps you to slow down and savor it.

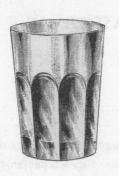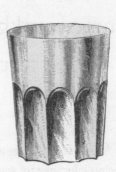

Buy smaller plates
and glasses.

The bigger the portion, the more we will eat—upward of 30 percent more. Food marketers know this, so they supersize our portions as a way to get us to buy more. But we don't have to supersize portions at home, and shouldn't. One researcher found that simply switching from a twelve-inch to a ten-inch dinner plate caused people to reduce their consumption by 22 percent.

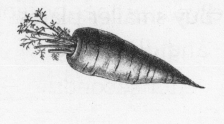

Serve a proper portion and don't go back for seconds.

You lose all control over portion size when you have second helpings. So what is a proper portion? There is folklore offering some sensible rules of thumb based on your size. One adage says you should never eat a portion of animal protein bigger than your fist. Another says that you should eat no more food at a meal than would fit into the bowl formed by your hands when cupped together. If you are going to break the rule on seconds, at least wait several minutes before doing it: You may well discover you don't really need seconds, or if you do, not as much as you thought.

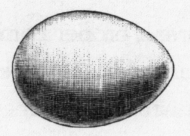

"Breakfast like a king, lunch like a prince, dinner like a pauper."

Eating a big meal late in the day sounds un-healthy, though in fact the science isn't conclusive. Some research suggests that eating close to bedtime elevates triglyceride levels in the blood, a marker for heart disease that is also implicated in weight gain. Also, the more physically active you are after a meal, the more of the energy in that meal your muscles will burn before your body stores it as fat. But some researchers believe a calorie is a calorie, no matter what time of day it is consumed. Even if this is true, however, front-loading your eating in the early part of the day will probably result in fewer total calories consumed, since people are generally less hungry in the morning. A related adage: "After lunch, sleep awhile; after dinner, walk a mile."

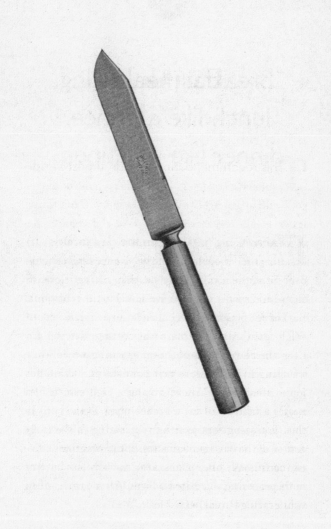

Eat meals.

This recommendation sounds almost as ridiculous as "eat food," but nowadays it too no longer goes without saying. We are snacking more and eating fewer meals together. Sociologists and market researchers who study American eating habits no longer organize their results around the increasingly quaint concept of the meal: They now measure "eating occasions" and report that we have added to the traditional Big Three—breakfast, lunch, and dinner—an as yet untitled fourth daily eating occasion that lasts all day long: the constant sipping and snacking we do while watching TV, driving, working, and so on. (One study found that among Americans ages eighteen to fifty nearly a fifth of all eating takes place in the car.) In theory, grazing—eating five or six small meals over the course of the day—makes sense, but in practice people eating this way often end up eating more, and eating more processed snack foods. So unless you can confine your grazing to real food, stick to meals.

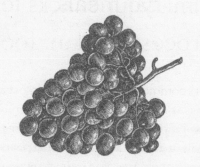

Limit your snacks to unprocessed plant foods.

Remember the old taboo against "between-meal snacks"? Decades of determined food marketing have driven the phrase from our consciousness. But the bulk of the 500 calories Americans have added to their daily diet since 1980 (the start of the obesity epidemic) have come in the form of snack foods laden with salt, fat, and sugar. If you are going to snack, try to limit yourself to fruits, vegetables, and nuts.

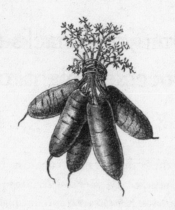

Don't get your fuel from the same place your car does.

American gas stations now make more money inside selling food (and cigarettes) than they do outside selling gasoline. But consider what kind of food this is: Except perhaps for the milk and water, it's all highly processed, imperishable snack foods and extravagantly sweetened soft drinks in hefty twenty-ounce bottles. Gas stations have become "processed corn stations": ethanol outside for your car and high-fructose corn syrup inside for you. Don't eat here.

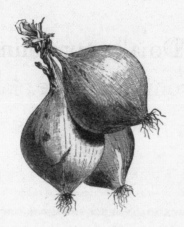

Do all your eating
at a table.

No, a desk is not a table. If we eat while we're working, or while watching TV or driving, we eat mindlessly—and as a result eat a lot more than we would if we were eating at a table, paying attention to what we're doing. This phenomenon can be tested (and put to good use): Place a child in front of a television set and place a bowl of fresh vegetables in front of him or her. The child will eat everything in the bowl, often even vegetables he or she doesn't ordinarily touch, without noticing what's going on. Which suggests an exception to the rule: When eating somewhere other than at a table, stick to fruits and vegetables.

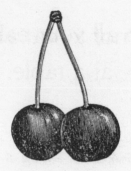

Try not to eat alone.

Americans are increasingly eating in soli-
tude. Although there is some research to suggest that light eaters will eat more when they dine with
others (perhaps because they spend more time at the
table), for people prone to overeating, communal meals
tend to limit consumption, if only because we're less
likely to stuff ourselves when others are watching. We
also tend to eat more slowly, since there's usually more
going on at the table than ingestion. This is precisely
why so much food marketing is designed to encourage
us to eat in front of the TV or in the car: When we eat
alone, we eat more. But regulating appetite is only part
of the story: The shared meal elevates eating from a biological process of fueling the body to a ritual of family
and community.

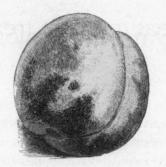

Treat treats as treats.

There is nothing wrong with special occasion foods, as long as every day is not a special occasion. This is another case where the outsourcing of our food preparation to corporations has gotten us into trouble: It's made formerly expensive or time-consuming foods—everything from fried chicken and french fries to pastries and ice cream—easy and readily accessible. Frying chicken is so much trouble that people didn't use to make it unless they had guests coming over and a lot of time to prepare. The amount of work involved kept the frequency of indulgence in check. These special occasion foods offer some of the great pleasures of life, so we shouldn't deprive ourselves of them, but the sense of occasion needs to be restored. One way is to start making these foods yourself; if you bake dessert yourself, you won't go to that much trouble every day. Another is to limit your consumption of such foods to weekends or social occasions. Some people follow a so-called S policy: "no snacks, no seconds, no sweets—except on days that begin with the letter S."

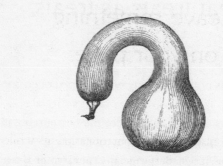

Leave something
on your plate.

Many of us were told by our parents while growing up that we should always clean our plates—an instruction that in later life we have perhaps taken a little too much to heart. But there is an older and healthier tradition that holds it is more genteel *not* to finish every last morsel of food: "Leave something for Mr. Manners," some children once were told, or, "Better to go to waste than to waist." Practice *not* cleaning your plate; it will help you eat less in the short term and develop self-control in the long.

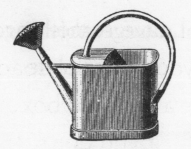

Plant a vegetable garden
if you have the space,
a window box
if you don't.

What does growing some of your own food have to do with repairing your relationship to food and eating? Everything. To take part in the intricate and endlessly interesting processes of providing for your sustenance is the surest way to escape the culture of fast food and the values implicit in it: that food should be fast, cheap, and easy; that food is a product of industry, not nature; that food is fuel rather than a form of communion with other people, and also with other species—with nature. On a more practical level, you will eat what your garden yields, which will be the freshest, most nutritious produce obtainable; you will get exercise growing it (and get outdoors and away from screens); you will save money (according to the National Gardening Association, a seventy-dollar investment in a vegetable garden will yield six hundred dollars' worth of food); and you will be that much more likely to follow the next, all-important rule.

Cook.

In theory, it should make little difference to your health whether you cook for yourself or let someone else do the work. But unless you can afford to hire a private chef to prepare meals exactly to your specifications, letting other people cook for you means losing control over your eating life, the portions as much as the ingredients. Cooking for yourself is the only sure way to take back control of your diet from the food scientists and food processors, and to guarantee you're eating real food and not edible foodlike substances, with their unhealthy oils, high-fructose corn syrup, and surfeit of salt. Not surprisingly, the decline in home cooking closely parallels the rise in obesity, and research suggests that people who cook are more likely to eat a more healthful diet.

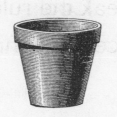

Break the rules
once in a while.

Obsessing over food rules is bad for your happiness, and probably for your health too. Our experience over the past few decades suggests that dieting and worrying too much about nutrition has made us no healthier or slimmer; cultivating a relaxed attitude toward food is important. There will be special occasions when you will want to throw these rules out the window. All will not be lost (especially if you don't throw out number 60). What matters is not the special occasion but the everyday practice—the default habits that govern your eating on a typical day. "All things in moderation," it is often said, but we should never forget the wise addendum, sometimes attributed to Oscar Wilde: "Including moderation."

Acknowledgments

I want to thank all the people who helped in the writing of this book, many of whom I don't know by name, and many of whom don't even know they've helped. But several I'm happy to be able to acknowledge by name. David Ludwig, MD, read the manuscript and made many valuable suggestions; he also caught several errors, though he shouldn't be held responsible for any that remain. He has been an invaluable teacher on questions of nutrition. So has Daphne Miller, MD, who contributed several memorable rules drawn from her medical practice and extensive fieldwork on traditional diets around the world. I've also learned a lot about diet and health from my conversations with Marion Nestle, Walter Willett, and Joan Gussow, even though I'm sure each will find things to disagree with in these pages. Special thanks to Tara Parker-Pope at the *New York Times* for letting me solicit rules on her blog, and to her readers, whose overwhelming response enriched the project immeasurably. My old friend and colleague Michael Schwarz read the manuscript and improved it with his editing; thank you once again. Thanks again, too, to Amanda Urban and her crack team at ICM, and to the wonderful crew at Penguin, but especially to Ann Godoff, Lindsay Whalen, Holly Watson, and Rachel Burd. For her first-rate research and editing I'm grateful to Malia Wollan. Adrienne Davich also contributed valuable research and fact-checking. And finally, heartfelt thanks to Judith and Isaac, the best dinner companions anyone could wish for; your ideas and words (not to mention your cooking) always nourish me, and particularly nourished this book.